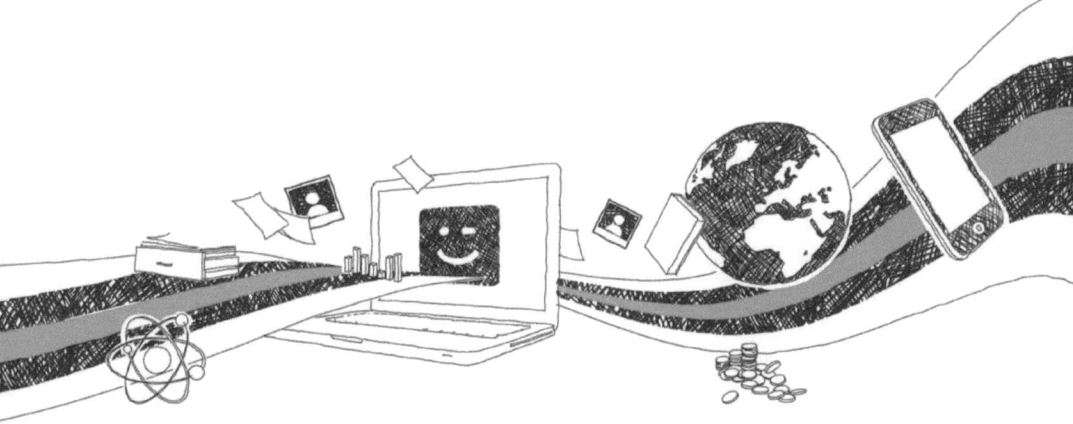
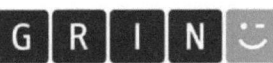

Bibliographic information published by the German National Library:

The German National Library lists this publication in the National Bibliography; detailed bibliographic data are available on the Internet at http://dnb.dnb.de .

Imprint:

Copyright © 2016 GRIN Verlag
Print and binding: Books on Demand GmbH, Norderstedt Germany
ISBN: 9783668613102

This book at GRIN:

https://www.grin.com/document/387175

Ratib Mawa

Area of residence and risk of cardiovascular disease and mortality among adults with type 1 diabetes mellitus in Stockholm County

A Swedish cohort study

GRIN Verlag

GRIN - Your knowledge has value

Since its foundation in 1998, GRIN has specialized in publishing academic texts by students, college teachers and other academics as e-book and printed book. The website www.grin.com is an ideal platform for presenting term papers, final papers, scientific essays, dissertations and specialist books.

Visit us on the internet:

http://www.grin.com/

http://www.facebook.com/grincom

http://www.twitter.com/grin_com

Department of Public Health Sciences
Master Programme in Public Health Sciences
Public Health Epidemiology
Degree Project, 30credits
Spring term 2016

Area of residence and risk of cardiovascular disease and mortality among adults with type 1 diabetes mellitus in Stockholm County. A Swedish cohort study.

Master thesis for Degree of Master of Medical Science (120 with a Major in Public Health Sciences

Author: Mawa Ratib
Date of submission: June 2, 2016

Department of Public Health Sciences
Master Programme in Public Health Sciences
Public Health Epidemiology
Degree Project, 30credits

Master in Public Health Sciences report series

The master education in public health at Karolinska Institutet is a collaborative work of mainly three departments: The department of public health sciences, the Department of Learning, Informatics, Management and Ethics and the Institute of Environmental Medicine.

Abstract

Background: Cardiovascular disease (CVD) remains a major public health problem in Sweden. Area of residence has been suggested to increase the risk of CVD and CVD specific mortality in the general population but less investigated in adults with type 1 diabetes mellitus.

Setting; Disadvantaged areas identified for metropolitan development initiative in 1998 were compared to other areas within the urban Swedish county of Stockholm.

Aim

To deepen knowledge on health inequalities at area level by assessing whether the risk of incident CVD and CVD specific mortality among adults with type 1 diabetes mellitus living in disadvantaged areas differed from those in other areas of Stockholm County.

Methods: A cohort study in which 7544 adults with type 1 diabetes mellitus aged 40-80 years, living in disadvantaged and other areas of Stockholm County in 2006 were followed from 2006-2011. Crude and adjusted hazard ratios for incident CVD and CVD specific mortality were calculated using Cox proportional hazard regression. All models were adjusted for age, gender, education, country of birth, social allowance, disability allowance and disposable income.

Results: Adjusted hazard ratios for CVD, stroke, peripheral vascular disease, myocardial infarction and CVD specific mortality were 1.2 (95% CI 0.5-2.0), 1.2 (95% CI 0.6-3.1), 1.0 (95% CI 0.5-2.9), 1.9 (95% CI 1.07-3.6) and 1.3 (95% CI 0.5-4.5) respectively for subjects in disadvantaged areas compared to other areas of Stockholm County.

Conclusion: Area of residence was not associated with incident CVD as composite endpoint, stroke, PVD and CVD specific mortality however an association with incident myocardial infarction was observed.

Keywords: Area of residence, cardiovascular disease, stroke, myocardial infarction, peripheral vascular disorders, mortality, morbidity.

Table of Contents

List of Abbreviations

CVD	Cardiovascular Disease
CHD	Coronary Heart Diseases
ICD	International Classification of Diseases
MI	Myocardial Infarction
OECD	Organisation for Economic Cooperation and Development
PVD	Peripheral Vascular Diseases
PIN	Personal Identification Number
T1DM	Type 1 Diabetes Mellitus
ITS	World Health Organisation

1 Background

According to the Institute of Health Matrix and the World Health Organisation (WHO), cardiovascular disease (CVD) remains the leading cause of non-communicable disease (NCD) morbidity and mortality in adults aged ≥ 30 years [1-3]. Although a considerable decline in global CVD morbidity and mortality especially in developed countries was registered in recent decades [2, 4, 5], in the year 2012, the WHO estimated that 17.5 million (37% of NCD) deaths in adults under 70 years of age were attributed to CVD [3] and case fatality is expected to rise to approximately 23.6 million by 2030 [6], making it a large scale global public health problem and underpins the need for increased public health efforts to combat its burden in society.

In Western Europe, Sweden is one of the countries with high CVD burden [7-9]. CVD accounted for 41% all cause mortality among adults aged 30-70 years in the year 2012 [10] and age- adjusted CVD death rates for men and women were 222.5 and 144.9 (per 100,000 people) respectively in 2010 [10]. This high burden of CVD was mainly attributed to the prevalence of biological and behavioural risk factors such as hypertension, smoking, physical inactivity etc [11-15] as well as surrogate contextual factors in the social and physical environments where people live and work, for instance socio-economic deprivation in area of residence [16-19]. However, interventions such as treatment with potent pharmacological drugs [20-22], surgical procedures e.g. vascularisation [23], dietary modifications [24, 25], increased physical activity [26, 27], tobacco control policies [28, 29] and control of hypertension and other risk factors [30, 31] have somewhat mitigated the high burden of CVD with notable decline in mortality due to stroke and coronary heart diseases reported in recent decades [16, 32, 33].

The WHO defined cardiovascular disease as a disorder of the blood vessels and the heart [6]. The main classifications and leading causes of CVD mortality and morbidity include coronary heart diseases (CHD), Cerebrovascular diseases, peripheral vascular diseases (PVD), deep venous thrombosis, hypertensive heart disease and inflammatory heart diseases as well as stroke and myocardial infarction which are some acute CVD events resulting mainly from impaired blood supply to the brain and myocardial tissues respectively. CVD exerts profound health, social and economic impact on individuals and societies. Apart from impairing quality of life and causing premature death [1, 9, 34], CVD incur enormous economic costs which exacerbate poverty and retards economic growth as a result of reduced labour force due to morbidity and premature deaths [34-36]. In the year 2009, the economic cost incurred to CVD in Sweden revealed non-health care costs of approximately €1.6 million (2% of the total health care expenditure) and direct health care costs of €2.4million equivalent to 8% of the national health care expenditure [37]. This is a huge amount of money that would have done enormous work if it were invested in other national development initiatives.

The major CVD risk factors are known, the challenge remains with reduction of their prevalence in various populations through promoting healthy lifestyles and health seeking behaviours in a life-course perspective [6]. The proximal CVD risk factors are either modifiable or non-modifiable. The most common modifiable risk factors include hypertension, tobacco use, diabetes, physical inactivity, unhealthy diet, high blood cholesterol level and overweight/obesity. The non-modifiable risk factors include age, gender and family history of CVD (19). Exposure to proximal CVD risk factors tends to be largely influenced by surrogate contextual risk factors in the social and physical environments in which people live and work [38, 39]. Social conditions in which people live and work commonly measured using socio-economic status at individual or area level has been well documented as a social determinant of CVD morbidity and mortality [40, 41]. These conditions are known to reflect access to resources such as health knowledge, money, power as well as prestige and social connections that are beneficial [40] and largely influence the distribution of the proximal biological and behavioural risk factors for CVD, consequentially leading to inequalities in CVD morbidity and mortality in the general population [39, 40] as theorised by Link and Phelan in 1995 when they illustrated that "social conditions are the fundamental causes of disease" in society [42].

More recently, Diez Roux illustrated pathways linking residential environments to CVD morbidity and mortality [43]   In their description, social factors in residential neighbourhoods such as violence and safety, social cohesion and support may influence coping mechanisms for CVD biological precursors such as stress. Social norms in area of residence may also lead to adoption of unhealthy behaviours such as poor dietary habits, physical inactivity and smoking which increase the risk of hypertension, obesity, diabetes and subsequently CVD. The physical environment in residential areas also plays a role in CVD causality. Components of residential area`s physical environment such as access to recreational resources, sidewalk ways, bike lanes, street connectivity, aesthetic quality, access to healthy foods, food and tobacco advertisement, availability of tobacco, noise and air pollution play a big role in influencing detrimental health behaviours such as smoking, physical inactivity, stress coping mechanisms, sleep disturbance etc which are known biological risk factors for CVD [38, 41, 43-47]. The above components of the social and physical environments of residential areas were postulated not to act in isolation but also

2

interact with each other resulting to potential multi-factorial causal network that link area of residence to CVD morbidity and mortality. This therefore underscores the role of residential areas in influencing inequalities in CVD risk and mortality and the need for it to be taken into consideration in the efforts to combat CVD morbidity and mortality.

Type 1 diabetes (T1DM) is a metabolic disorder which commonly occurs in children but also in adults. It occurs as a result of cell-mediated autoimmune destruction of the pancreatic beta-cells resulting into insulin deficiency, failure of blood glucose regulation and subsequently a myriad of complications [48]. It accounts for 5-10 % of all diabetes cases [48, 49]. Time trend analysis from 1983-2007 showed an increasing incidence of T1DM in young Swedish population aged 0-34years and it has been ranked as the 12th leading cause of mortality and morbidity in the globe in the year 2010 [50, 51]. T1DM is also a risk factor for CVD, making patients with this condition more susceptible to CVD than the general population as described by de Ferranti et al in their recent systematic review [49]. Similarly some recent studies in Sweden have shown that the incidence of CVD in adults with T1DM is on rise [52, 53]. Simultaneous exposure to other proximal CVD risk factors will increase CVD risk profile and the probability of developing CVD among adults with T1DM [1, 49, 54] and yet the combined effect of CVD [55] and myriad of other complications in T1DM patients is demanding and requires regular contact with medical doctors / health care facilities [56]. Effective control of other CVD risk factors and a functional high quality and accessible health care is therefore paramount to prolong and improve quality of life and reduce inequalities in CVD morbidity and mortality in adults with T1DM.

More encouraging is the equitable access to high quality health care and good performance of the Swedish health care system in comparison to other countries of the Organisation for Economic Cooperation and Development (OECD) in recent decades [57]. However, social differentials were suggested to be widening and isolated issues of access especially with regards to specialists care waiting time, rural-urban differences and user fee are still prevalent [58-61]. Critiques also argue that the recent changes in Swedish welfare state arrangements [61] and the shift to the market oriented healthcare [62] which might have resulted into withdrawal of extra resources from primary health care in disadvantaged areas [63] may likely favour socially advantaged groups and could further increase health and social inequalities [61, 64, 65]. CVD remains a major public health problem in Sweden as alluded to earlier on [66], its prevention and control is therefore a public health priority and essential for achievement of national public health targets and the realization of the WHO goal of reducing non-communicable diseases burden by 25% by 2025 [1, 67].

3

Targeting CVD vulnerable populations is therefore an important public health prevention strategy.

Although area disadvantage has been shown to increase the risk of CVD and CVD mortality in the general population, studies in adults with T1DM are rare to find in published literature. This study therefore aimed to deepen knowledge on residential area inequalities in CVD morbidity and mortality among adults with T1DM in Stockholm County. The expectation was that the risk of incident CVD and CVD specific mortality would be higher in adults with T1DM living in disadvantaged areas compared to other areas of Stockholm County. The study's significance lies in adding to the growing knowledge of the residential area inequalities in the risk of incident CVD and CVD mortality in adults with T1DM and the award of my degree of masters in public health epidemiology. The findings may be of value to public health practitioners interested in designing targeted CVD prevention and control interventions and could also inform re-shaping of CVD prevention and control policies/strategies by public health policy makers in Stockholm County.

1.1 Area of residence

Area of residence intrinsically embodies components of the social and physical environment that influence health as described earlier on [38, 43]. Area disadvantage commonly referred to as area deprivation is a widely used concept with no single definition [68]. Some social epidemiologists claimed that it summarizes an area's health risk potential based on geographical clustering of unemployment, poverty, social disorganization and economic divesture [69]. The choice of area of residence is influenced by several factors among which socio-economic status and culture play key role [40, 70]. A number of countries developed indices of area deprivation/disadvantage that suits the ecological characteristics of their populations. These indices remain the most widely used measures for assessing residential area inequalities in health and disease [71, 72]. Examples include the Swedish Care Need Index [73] and the English Index of Multiple Deprivation [74]. However in this study, we did not use deprivation index but rather dichotomised individuals into either disadvantaged or other areas of Stockholm County based on classification of residential areas in Stockholm County in 1998 for metropolitan development initiative[75]

1.2 Area of residence and risk of CVD in adults with T1DM

Published longitudinal studies consistently showed increased risk of myocardial infarction[18, 76-78], coronary heart disease[46, 79, 80],stroke[81, 82], CVD [43, 82] and peripheral vascular diseases [83] among residents of disadvantaged areas compared to

4

least disadvantaged areas in the general population. In most of these studies, after adjusting for contextual and individual level covariates, the effect remained, implying existence of an independent association between residential area disadvantage and CVD. However whether this association is causal is still a matter of debate as many critiques argue that limited empirical evidence exists to explain how residential area disadvantage can influence biological mechanisms for development of CVD. Presence of residual confounding and possible interaction of contextual factors in area of residence were some of the alternative explanations that might not be ruled out, given the use of different composite deprivation indices often derived from individual level risk factors [44, 68] as well as the possibility that the observed association between area of residence and risk of CVD might reflect the effect of risk accumulation over life-course [43, 45]. Though widely investigated in the general population, the association between area of residence and risk of incident CVD has been less investigated in subjects with T1DM who are more vulnerable to CVD than people without diabetes. Area deprivation is therefore more likely to increase their vulnerability, reduce their quality of life and chances of survival.

A cross-sectional study conducted in France found a 4-fold increase in the risk of retinopathy in more deprived patients compared to the least deprived [84].Rawshani et al in a 6-year follow-up cohort study in Sweden also found that individuals in the lowest income quintiles had 2-fold increase in the risk of non-fatal/fatal CVD event, coronary heart disease and stroke when compared to those in the highest income quintile [17]. These few studies point to the importance of socio-economic deprivation in relation to CVD risk and may therefore be important to conduct more studies to demonstrate the consistency and temporality of this association relevant for causality judgment and making evidence based decisions by public health policy makers and practitioners for targeted CVD prevention and control interventions.

1.3 Area of residence and risk of cardiovascular disease specific mortality in adults with T1DM

A systematic review by Matteucci and Giampietro showed that adults with T1DM had 2-4 fold increase in CVD mortality when compared to the general population[85]. A longitudinal study from the UK that assessed the effect of material deprivation measured using the Townsend scores found an increased risk of CVD specific mortality among subjects with T1DM aged ≤35years. Those with the highest score of material deprivation had age standardised mortality ratio and 95% confidence interval of 1365 (727 to 2334) for female and 536 (332 to 819) for men[86]. A similar study among T1DM patients aged 17-65years also found an increased risk of CVD mortality in socio-economically deprived adults compared to those in higher social class; Odds Ratio 3.98 (95% CI 1.96-8.06) and a

6-fold increased risk of CVD mortality among the unemployed compared to the employed[87]. Likewise, a more recent Swedish study also found a socio-economic gradient in the risk of CVD mortality among subjects with T1DM[88].Although these studies have inherent weakness, especially with regards to statistical adjustment for contextual and some individual level risk factors, they still provide plausible explanation of material deprivation/socio-economic status (key components of social and physical environment of area of residence) as predictors of CVD specific mortality in this group of patients. Given the myriad of other medical complications experienced by patients with T1DM, their health and medical care needs surpass those of the general population. Therefore ascertaining residential area inequalities in CVD specific mortality in subjects with T1DM is essential for planning targeted CVD preventions and control interventions and policy modifications. Overall, previous studies consistently showed that material deprivation and socio-economic status often linked to area of residence is associated with increased risk of CVD and CVD specific mortality.

2 Aim and research questions

2.1 Aim

To deepen knowledge on health inequalities at area level by assessing whether the risk of incident CVD and CVD specific mortality among adults with type 1 diabetes mellitus living in disadvantaged areas differed from those in other area of residence in Stockholm County.

2.2 Research Questions

The following research questions were answered in this study.

1. Is there difference in the risk of incident CVD among adults with T1DM living in disadvantaged areas compared to other areas of Stockholm county?
2. Does the risk of incident CVD types; myocardial infarction (MI), stroke, and peripheral vascular disease (PVD) differ among adults with type 1 diabetes mellitus living in disadvantaged areas compared to other areas of Stockholm County?
3. Is there difference in the risk of CVD specific mortality among adults with T1DM living in disadvantaged areas compared to other areas of Stockholm county?

3 Materials and methods

3.1 Study design and population

A register based Swedish cohort study in which 12709 adults with T1DM living in Stockholm County in 2006 were identified from the Swedish prescribed drug register. After excluding 4612 subjects who were either ≤ 40 or ≥ 80 years of age and 553 subjects who had experienced CVD event by 31st December 2005, our study base consisted of 7544 (4327 male and 3217 female) subjects with T1DM aged 40-80years, who were followed from 1st January 2006 to 31st December 2011 for the outcomes of interest. A cohort study design was chosen because of our interest in incident CVD events and cumulative hazard over 6-year period to estimate relative risk differences for incident CVD and CVD specific mortality among adults with T1DM living in disadvantaged verses other areas of Stockholm county.

3.2 Data Sources

Data was obtained from four Swedish registers. These included the Swedish Prescribed Drug Register, the National Inpatient Register, Cause of Death Register and the Integrated Database for Labour Market Research register (LISA). These registers are managed by Statistics Sweden, the legally mandated custodian of 119 official national statistics registers in Sweden [89].

The Swedish Prescribed Drug Register

Subjects with T1DM were identified from this newly established register of the National Board of Health and Welfare of Sweden. Information recorded in this register included; patient's unique identifier, age in years, gender, diagnosis and the prescribers profession and/or area of specialization[90].

The Swedish Inpatient Register

Started in 1964, each hospital case diagnosis and discharge are keyed to individual patient's morbidity record through personal identification number- PIN [91]. Cases of first event of CVD were recorded and retrieved based on the International Statistical Classification of Disease and related health problem (ICD-10) codes. The inpatient register has high validity [92].

The Swedish Cause of death registers

T1DM patients were followed for CVD specific mortality through this register. All cases of death in Sweden are recorded in the cause of death register since 1961[93]. From 1997, case diagnosis and deaths were recorded based on ICD-10; the same was for retrieval of data on CVD specific deaths for this study. This register was also known to have high validity [93].

Integrated Database for Labour Market Research (LISA)

Subjects with T1DM were linked to LISA using their anonymous PIN to obtain individual information on area of residence, gainful employment, income from gainful employment, income from social assistance, occupational pension, unemployment benefits, country of birth and parental countries of birth, year of migration, place of employment and education level.

3.3 Study setting

In 1998 the Swedish government through the ministry of Labour conducted a survey in major cities of Sweden to identify socio-economically vulnerable populations and their areas of residence[75]. In Stockholm County, sixteen areas were identified and categorised as disadvantaged areas based on three parameters; high proportion of foreign-born people, high levels of unemployment and high proportion of people with low level of education. These areas included; Husby, Rinkeby, Rågsved, Skärholmen, Tensta, Alby, Fittja, Hallunda-Norsborg, Jordbro, Flemingsberg, Vårby, VästraSkogås, Fornhöjden, Geneta, Hovsjö, and Ronna. The same year, a metropolitan development initiative was then launched in all major cities aimed to reduce segregation and improve the living standards of vulnerable populations. In this study, we used area of residence described in the metropolitan development initiative in 1998 to identify adults with T1DM living in the above sixteen disadvantaged areas of Stockholm county in 2006 and compared them with respect to outcomes of interest to those with T1DM living in other areas of the county.

3.4 Exposure

Area of residence in Stockholm County in 2006 was the exposure of interest in this study. The Swedish personal identification number was used to identify study subject's area of residence through data linkage to LISA. Study subjects were grouped into two areas of residence classified as disadvantaged and other areas of Stockholm County based on proportions of foreign born people, the unemployed and level of education. A disadvantaged area was defined as areas with high levels of unemployment, foreign born residents and people with low level of education. Other areas of Stockholm County included those with relatively low levels of unemployment, foreign born people and those with low level of education. More information about these parameters has already been described elsewhere[75] and the exposure definition as used in this study has been utilised in some other studies [94, 95].

3.5 Covariates

Age, gender, education and socio-economic status have been associated with increased risk of CVD and CVD mortality in published literature [96, 97]. Based on their availability

8

in the dataset and literature information we included the variables described below as confounders not ruling out the possibility that they could act as mediators in the relationship between area of residence and the outcomes of interest in this study, especially in the case of education and income. **Age**: was recorded and retrieved in years and used as a categorical variable. Four age groups of ten year interval were created; 40-49, 50-59, 60-69 and 70-80 years. **Gender** was recorded as male and female in the registers and used as a dichotomous variable. **Education**: was recorded and retrieved as primary, secondary and specific post-secondary professional qualifications. Subjects were then grouped into those with primary (9-10 years of schooling), secondary (at least 1 year secondary school) and Post-secondary school (at least 1 years of post-secondary education).**Social allowance**: In Sweden, social allowance is provided to people who are unemployed or who have lost their jobs once they notify the government about their employment status. Study subjects were grouped into those who were either receiving or not receiving social allowance in 2006 based. **Disability pension**: This is normally provided to people who have experienced any kind of disability that prevent them from working for paid jobs. Participants were grouped into those on disability pension, not on disability pension and retired persons not entitle to disability pension. **Disposable income**: was recorded and retrieved in Swedish Kronor. Income quintiles were then developed; subjects were grouped into five income quintiles based on their level of income. Data on the socio-demographic characteristics was obtained from LISA, inpatient and cause of death registers as described earlier on. **Country of birth:** Due to the small number of cases, we grouped country of birth into five regions; Africa, Asia, Sweden, Europe and OECD together, and Latin America.

3.6 Outcomes

The outcomes investigated in this study were; Incident CVD as composite endpoint, stroke, myocardial infarction (MI) peripheral vascular disease (PVD) and CVD specific mortality based on Swedish inpatient and cause of death registers data. These outcomes were defined as defined as ICD-10; Myocardial infarction: I2100 to I2299, Cerebrovascular diseases: I6000 to I6499 and Arteries, arterioles, capillaries and peripheral circulatory complications: E105, E115, E125, E135, E145, and I7000 to I7999 respectively. All data regarding inpatient diagnosis of CVD and CVD death for each study subject with T1DM were available in the inpatient and cause of death register respectively. Before analysis of the data Subjects with T1DM in 2006 were linked to the available inpatient register data from 2000 until 2011. Individuals with previous CVD diagnosis in the inpatient register from 2000 to 2005 were excluded from the analysis in order to include and analyse only incident cases of CVD and CVD specific mortality. To ensure

9

individuals with T1DM appear once in the count of incident CVD and CVD specific mortality, serial numbers that replaced the patient PIN were used for data linkage across registers. Subjects were followed from 1st Jan 2006 when CVD free through 31st December 2011. Follow-up ended when a study subject developed incident CVD, died, migrated out of Stockholm County or reached the end of study period in 2011 without experiencing CVD event. Those who died due to a cause other than CVD, migrated out of Stockholm County or did not develop CVD at end of the study period were right censored in the analysis.

4 Statistical analysis

Although the most recommended statistical modelling method to employ for analysing hierarchical data would have been multilevel modelling, the small sample size and the number of fatal and non-fatal CVD events in some residential areas would have led to unreliable estimates of the effect measures, let alone our interest in macro-level residential area differences in the risk of incident CVD and CVD specific mortality. To determine whether subjects differed with regards to the distribution of potential confounding variables, we used descriptive analysis to compare baseline socio-demographic characteristics of the study subjects with respect to area of residence. Chi-square test at 5% level of significance was used test differences in distribution of the categorical variables. Data exploration in the primary analysis revealed one covariate (education level) with 1% of the study subjects missing values. Incidence rates based on person years as denominator were used in the computation of the hazard ratios. To calculate the hazard ratios (HR) for incident CVD, stroke, MI, PVD and CVD specific deaths, we first conducted univariate analysis to determine covariates that were associated with each of the above outcomes. Cox proportional hazard analysis was then used to calculate the 6-year period crude and adjusted hazard ratios with the 95% confidence intervals for incident CVD, MI, stroke, PVD and CVD specific mortality for adults with T1DM living in disadvantaged areas compared to other areas of Stockholm county. The proportional hazard assumption for each of the outcomes by area of residence in the six year period was assessed by plotting the Kaplan-Meier curves. Crude and adjusted models were developed for each outcome to compare the risk of the outcomes of interest among T1DM living in disadvantaged verses other areas of Stockholm county. All covariates described above were adjusted for in each model during the analysis. Using step-wise covariate selection method, the resulting model for each outcome contained area of residence, age and gender, however coefficients for age and gender were not reported as this was not the objective of this study. Analysis was performed with the aid of Statistical Analysis System software – SAS version 9.4.

10

5 Ethical Considerations

This research was not conducted among vulnerable population groups, but use of study subjects personal identification number could present potential harm to study subjects as a result of access to sensitive personal information. To protect their privacy, the Swedish personal identification numbers [91] were replaced with anonymous numbers which did not allow identification of individual data. Another ethical concern was the issue of informed consent given the use of registers based data. Even though obtaining informed consent from study subjects was not done, the Swedish personal data act provides safeguard for subject's personal data and confidentiality [98]. Measures were also taken to prevent access to the research data by unauthorized persons through restricting data analysis and storage to protected institutional office computer of Karolinska Institutet.

To enhance validity of the findings, appropriate study design and study population were chosen. Data from the high quality Swedish registers were used and appropriate statistical analysis techniques applied to estimate effect measures. Known and accessible confounders and other covariates were controlled for to exclude other alternative explanations for residential area differences in the risk of incident CVD and CVD specific mortality. This study had potential benefits to individuals and the Swedish society. The findings could influence individuals with T1DM to engage in health seeking behaviors that may help reduce their future risk of CVD and mortality. Society may also benefit through use of the results by health policy makers to re-shape CVD prevention and control policies for reduction of residential area inequalities in CVD morbidity and mortality. Lastly the findings could also provide a hint to public health practitioners when making choice for target populations to be included in interventions intended to reduce CVD mortality and morbidity in Stockholm County. The researcher has no conflict of interest related to undertaking this study. This study was vetted and approved by the Regional Ethical Review Board for Stockholm County (Dnr 2013/1268-31/4).

6 Results

6.1 Socio-demographic characteristics of adults with type 1 diabetes mellitus

Table 1 shows the baseline socio-demographic characteristics of T1DM cohort according to area of residence in Stockholm County in 2006. Subjects with T1DM living in disadvantaged areas had similar age-group distribution to those in other areas of Stockholm County. However differences were apparent with regards to gender, education, income, social allowance and disability pension. More men than women, fewer T1DM patients with post secondary education, those in high income group and majority of those on social allowance and disability pension lived in disadvantaged areas compared to other areas of Stockholm County.

6.2 Risk of incident CVD, stroke, myocardial infarction and peripheral vascular disease according to area of residence.

During the 6-year follow-up period, 306 cases of incident CVD occurred among the 7544 adults with T1DM as shown in table 2. Subjects with T1DM living in disadvantaged areas compared to other areas were relatively high risk for all the outcomes. With exception of myocardial infarction, all incident CVD, stroke and PVD did not show statistical significance. After adjusting for age, gender, education, country of birth, social and disability allowance (Table 2), area of residence had no effect on the risk of incident CVD stroke, PVD though a slight reduction in the hazard ratio was observed. The hazard ratio for incident MI for subjects with T1DM living in disadvantaged areas compared to other areas of Stockholm county slightly increased and remained marginally significant.

6.3 Risk of CVD specific mortality according to area of residence

After the 6-year follow-up period, 551 all cause deaths were registered, of these 54 were due to CVD and 497 due to other causes. As shown in table 3, the crude hazard ratio for CVD specific mortality was 1.6, which attenuated to 1.3 after adjusting for age, gender, education, individual income, social allowance and disability allowance.

Table 1 Socio-demographic characteristics of (N= 7544) adults with type 1 diabetes mellitus according to area of residence in Stockholm County in 2006.

	AREA OF RESIDENCE		
Variables	**Disadvantaged**	**Other areas**	
	n (%)	n (%)	**P-value**
Gender			
Male	292 (53)	4035 (58)	<0.05
Female	262 (47)	2955 (42)	
Age in years			
40-49	142 (26)	1738 (25)	0.17
50-59	168 (30)	1867 (27)	
60-69	136 (24)	1956 (28)	
70-80	108 (20)	1429 (20)	
Education			
Low (Primary)	219 (43)	1783 (26)	<0.01
Medium (Secondary)	199 (39)	2997 (43)	
High(Post-secondary)	91 (18)	2144 (31)	
Individual income Quintiles			
1(Lowest)	159 (29)	963 (14)	<0.01
2	162 (29)	1471 (22)	
3	116 (21)	1504 (21)	
4	78 (14)	1482 (21)	
5(Highest)	39 (7)	1570 (22)	
Social Allowance			
Not receiving	446 (81)	6724 (96)	<0.01
Receiving	108 (19)	266 (4)	
Disability pension			
Not receiving	257 (46)	3666 (52)	<0.01
Receiving	142 (26)	1280 (18)	
Retired	155 (28)	2044 (30)	
Country of birth			
Africa	41 (7)	120 (2)	<0.01
Asia	158 (29)	269 (4)	
Sweden	229(41)	5671 (81)	
Europe and OECD	97(18)	779 (11)	
Latin America	29 (5)	151 (2)	

Missing Values: Education = 45 subjects living in disadvantaged areas and 66 in other areas of Stockholm

Table 2 Crude and adjusted hazard ratios for incident CVD, stroke, peripheral vascular disease and myocardial infarction according to area of residence in a cohort of (N=7544)adults with type 1 diabetes mellitus aged 40-80 years in Stockholm County, 2006-2011.

Area of residence	No. exposed	No. cases	Crude HR (95% CI)	Adjusted HR (95% CI)
All CVD				
Other areas	6990	272	1	1
Disadvantaged	554	34	1.3 (0.9-2.0)	1.2 (0.5-2.0)
Myocardial Infarction				
Other areas	6798	80	1	1
Disadvantaged	534	14	1.8 (1.0-3.4)	1.9 (1.1-3.6)[*]
Stroke				
Other areas	6823	95	1	1
Disadvantaged	530	10	1.3 (0.6-2.8)	1.2 (0.6-3.2)
Peripheral Vascular disease				
Other areas	6825	97	1	1
Disadvantaged	530	10	1.1 (0.5-2.5)	1.0 (0.5-2.9)

HR indicates Hazard Ratio; CI, Confidence Interval. Models for all outcomes were adjusted for age, gender, education, individual income, social allowance and disability allowance and country of birth.
[*] Statistically significant association.

Table 3 Crude and adjusted hazard ratios for CVD specific mortality according to area of residence in a cohort of (N=7544) adults with type 1 diabetes mellitus aged 40-80 years in Stockholm County, 2006-2011.

Area of residence	No. exposed	No. cases	Crude HR (95% CI)	Adjusted HR (95% CI)
All CVD				
Other areas	6470	44	1	1
Disadvantaged	523	10	1.6 (0.7-3.7)	1.3 (0.5-4.5)

HR indicates Hazard Ratio; CI, Confidence Interval. Adjusted for age, gender, education, individual income, Country of birth, social and disability allowance

7. Discussion

The present study suggests that area of residence is not associated with increased risk of incident CVD, stroke, PVD and CVD specific mortality in subjects with T1DM aged 40-80 years. Adjusting for confounders such as age, country of birth, education, social allowance, disability pension and gender in each of the models for the above outcomes would have controlled their effect which in-turn would have been reflected in observable changes in the effect measures, but this was not the case in this study given that the relationship between area of residence at baseline and the risk of incident CVD, stroke, PVD and CVD specific mortality did not change. These results are not in-line with those from previous studies that showed an increased risk of non-fatal CVD[17] and fatal CVD events[86, 87]. These could be attributed to relatively shorter follow-up time and study power that could have possibly hindered observation of more fatal and non-fatal CVD events given the nature of long induction period for CVD[99]. Although our study did not examine the effect of specific contextual factors in area of residence but rather the macro-level effects, one could advance the notion that excellent urban design of Stockholm County with walking/running lanes, bicycle lanes and the availability and access to other sports facilities provides equal opportunity to engage in physical activity and could partially explain the indifference in incident CVD, stroke and PVD with respect to area of residence. On the same note, the equity based Swedish health care system that allows equal access to care [100, 101] and the probable effect of the metropolitan development initiative that was aimed at reducing segregation and improving the living conditions of people in disadvantaged areas in major Swedish cities including Stockholm county might have also influenced the relationship between area of residence and the risk of incident CVD, stroke, PVD and CVD mortality[102]. Other explanations could be possibility of effective tobacco use policies[103] and alcohol consumption control policies[104, 105] and other public health policies for control of modifiable CVD risk factors in Sweden[106, 107].

Another important secondary finding in this study was that area of residence was associated with incident MI. This finding is in-line with the study by Rawshani et al [17]which showed a 2-fold increase in the risk of incident CVD including MI among T1DM patients in most deprived income group compared to those who were least deprived.MI is one of the earliest manifestations of CVD. The fact that MI tends to precede other types of incident CVD events investigated in this study could explain why this association was significant in our study. The increased risk of incident MI among subjects with T1DM living in disadvantaged areas might suggest the undesirable socio-economic impacts of the recent changes in the Swedish welfare state arrangements on the ability of adults with T1DM to meet their basic needs, possibly resulting to increased stress and unhealthy behaviours such as smoking, poor dietary habits etc. Secondly the shift to the market oriented health care which might have resulted into withdrawal of extra resources from primary health care in disadvantaged areas could have reduced access to health care services by adults with T1DM in disadvantaged areas. One could also assert that there might have been higher prevalence of probable unmeasured proximal biological and behavioural risk factors for MI among subjects with T1DM living in disadvantaged areas, given evidence of socio-economic gradient in the prevalence of established MI risk factors from longitudinal studies, let alone risk accumulation in a life-course perspective. On the other hand, cultural norms in areas of residence for example behaviours such as smoking, alcohol consumption could be more prevalent in disadvantaged areas and might influence adoption by non-practitioners as coping mechanism for stress resulting to MI risk factor accumulation. Given the volume of possible factors influencing MI development in area of residence, several pathways might be involved as well as the interactions of contextual and individual level risk factors.

8 Strengths and limitations

As earlier on stated, though the most appropriate statistical analysis method to employ for modelling a hierarchical data would have been multilevel modelling to account for the effect of both contextual and individual level confounding variables, few numbers of subjects with T1DM in higher level unit would have led to unreliable estimates. Using single level model might have as well underestimated the standard errors and resulted into narrow confidence intervals and increased probability of type 1 error. Secondly we did not have information about study subject's outpatient treatment/diagnosis making it probable that patients who might have had milder forms of CVD events could have been included in the study. Thirdly our results could have also been influenced by unknown confounders not adjusted for in the analysis, given the multi-factorial nature of CVD causal mechanism and the possibility of interactions that would increase the risk of incident CVD and CVD specific mortality at area level. Fourthly the reality that people change their areas of residence over the course of time might have led to non-differential misclassification of the outcome with respect to the exposure which might have biased the hazard ratios towards the null. Lastly use of T1DM patient's data for Stockholm County only makes it unlikely to generalise the results of this study to other T1DM patients in other parts of Sweden and developed countries with similar contexts. Despite of these weaknesses, our study also had strengths. First we used data from the high quality Swedish national registers that has high internal and external validity[92]. Secondly, there are no known studies to us that assessed residential area disparities in incident CVD risk and mortality among adults with T1DM in Stockholm County, this study is therefore one of the first if any and would provide the bases for more studies in the subject matter.

9 Conclusion and implications

Area of residence was not associated with incident CVD as a composite endpoint, stroke, PVD and CVD specific mortality however an association with incident myocardial infarction was observed. These results should however be interpreted with caution as it might reflect effect of unknown and uncontrolled confounders at contextual and individual level. Nevertheless public health policy makers and public health practitioners in Stockholm County may need to take into consideration residential area disadvantage when re-shaping policies and planning targeted public health interventions to reduce inequalities in future occurrence of myocardial infarction among adults with T1DM. Undertaking further rigorous studies with relatively larger sample size and longer follow-up period is essential as well as studies to explicate specific contextual factors that could be influencing inequalities in risk of incident CVD and CVD specific mortality among subjects with T1DM in Stockholm County might help shade more light.

10 Acknowledgment

My first thanks goes to Almighty God for the blessing of good health throughout the period of my thesis work. My mother Felister Limiyo, Father Ali Lomure Abdalla and beloved son Barack Emmanuel for enduring two years of my physical absence from home. Importantly this work has been a result of the support and encouragement from my supervisor and members of Karolinska Institutet equity and health policy research team. Thank you all for the inspiration, direct and indirect contributions throughout the period of my thesis work.

Dr Edison Manrique-Garcia, my outstanding supervisor. I would like to express my sincere gratitude for your continuous support, motivation, patience and immense knowledge, without which I wouldn't have made it to the end of this work. Thank you very much and may the Almighty God bless you abundantly.

Professor Bo Burström, Leader of research group on equity and health policy research for your invaluable input and encouragement. Your feedback on gaps in various sections of my thesis helped a lot in making the changes that improved the quality of my thesis.

Equity and Health Policy Research Team Members, Last but not least my sincere thanks also go to all distinguished researchers in the equity and health policy research team. Your guidance, encouragement and thought provoking questions helped me to reflect on the gaps that existed, improved my confidence and self-believe.

The Swedish Institute Scholarship; Lastly and most importantly my sincere thanks and gratitude goes to the Swedish Government especially to the Swedish Institute scholarship board for the scholarship award I received which provided the financial support I needed throughout my two year study program in Karolinska Institutet.

11 Reference

1. Roth GA, Huffman MD, Moran AE, Feigin V, Mensah GA, Naghavi M, Murray CJ: **Global and Regional Patterns in Cardiovascular Mortality From 1990 to 2013**. *Circulation* 2015, **132**(17):1667-1678.
2. Naghavi M, Wang H, Lozano R, Davis A, Liang X, Zhou M, Vollset SE, Ozgoren AA, Abdalla S, Abd-Allah F: **Global, regional, and national age-sex specific all-cause and cause-specific mortality for 240 causes of death, 1990-2013: a systematic analysis for the Global Burden of Disease Study 2013**. *Lancet* 2015, **385**(9963):117-171.
3. Mendis S: **Global Status Report on noncommunicable diseases 2014**. In. Geneva: WHO; 2014: 302.
4. Moran AE, Forouzanfar MH, Roth G, Mensah G, Ezzati M, Murray CJ, Naghavi M: **Temporal trends in ischemic heart disease mortality in 21 world regions, 1980-2010: The Global Burden of Disease 2010 Study**. *Circulation* 2014:CIRCULATIONAHA. 113.004042.
5. Berg J, Björck L, Lappas G, O'Flaherty M, Capewell S, Rosengren A: **Continuing decrease in coronary heart disease mortality in Sweden**. *BMC cardiovascular disorders* 2014, **14**(1):1.
6. Mendis S, Puska P, Norrving B: **Global atlas on cardiovascular disease prevention and control**: World Health Organization; 2011.
7. Nichols M, Townsend N, Scarborough P, Rayner M: **Cardiovascular disease in Europe: epidemiological update**. *European heart journal* 2013, **34**(39):3028-3034.
8. Linell A, Richardson MX, Wamala S: **The Swedish national public health policy report 2010**. *Scandinavian journal of public health* 2013, **41**(10 suppl):3-56.
9. Nichols M, Townsend N, Scarborough P, Rayner M: **European cardiovascular disease statistics 4th edition 2012: EuroHeart II**. *Eur Heart J* 2013, **34**(39):3007.
10. Nichols M, Townsend N, Scarborough P, Rayner M: **Cardiovascular disease in Europe 2014: epidemiological update**. *European heart journal* 2014:ehu299.
11. Conroy R, Pyörälä K, Fitzgerald Ae, Sans S, Menotti A, De Backer G, De Bacquer Dr, Ducimetiere P, Jousilahti P, Keil U: **Estimation of ten-year risk of fatal cardiovascular disease in Europe: the SCORE project**. *European heart journal* 2003, **24**(11):987-1003.
12. De Backer G, Ambrosionie E, Borch-Johnsen K, Brotons C, Cifkova R, Dallongeville J, Ebrahim S, Faergeman O, Graham I, Mancia G: **European guidelines on cardiovascular disease prevention in clinical practice: third joint task force of European and other societies on cardiovascular disease prevention in clinical practice (constituted by representatives of eight societies and by invited experts)**. *European Journal of Cardiovascular Prevention & Rehabilitation* 2003, **10**(1 suppl):S1-S78.
13. Yusuf S, Reddy S, Ôunpuu S, Anand S: **Global burden of cardiovascular diseases part I: general considerations, the epidemiologic transition, risk factors, and impact of urbanization**. *Circulation* 2001, **104**(22):2746-2753.
14. Ström J, Tavosian A, Appelros P: **Cardiovascular risk factors and TIA characteristics in 19,872 Swedish TIA patients**. *Acta Neurologica Scandinavica* 2016.
15. Vassilaki M, Linardakis M, Polk DM, Philalithis A: **The burden of behavioral risk factors for cardiovascular disease in Europe. A significant prevention deficit**. *Preventive medicine* 2015, **81**:326-332.
16. Nichols M, Townsend N, Scarborough P, Rayner M: **European cardiovascular disease statistics**; 2012.

17. Rawshani A, Svensson A-M, Rosengren A, Eliasson B, Gudbjörnsdottir S: **Impact of Socioeconomic Status on Cardiovascular Disease and Mortality in 24,947 Individuals With Type 1 Diabetes.** *Diabetes care* 2015:dc150145.

18. Stjärne MK, Diderichsen F, Reuterwall C, Hallqvist J: **Socioeconomic context in area of living and risk of myocardial infarction: results from Stockholm Heart Epidemiology Program (SHEEP).** *Journal of epidemiology and community health* 2002, **56**(1):29-35.

19. Sundquist K, Winkleby M, Ahlén H, Johansson S-E: **Neighborhood socioeconomic environment and incidence of coronary heart disease: a follow-up study of 25,319 women and men in Sweden.** *American journal of epidemiology* 2004, **159**(7):655-662.

20. Investigators FS: **Effects of long-term fenofibrate therapy on cardiovascular events in 9795 people with type 2 diabetes mellitus (the FIELD study): randomised controlled trial.** *The Lancet* 2005, **366**(9500):1849-1861.

21. Group SSSS: **Randomised trial of cholesterol lowering in 4444 patients with coronary heart disease: the Scandinavian Simvastatin Survival Study (4S).** *The Lancet* 1994, **344**(8934):1383-1389.

22. Kotseva K, Wood D, De Backer G, De Bacquer D, Pyörälä K, Keil U, Group ES: **EUROASPIRE III: a survey on the lifestyle, risk factors and use of cardioprotective drug therapies in coronary patients from 22 European countries.** *European Journal of Cardiovascular Prevention & Rehabilitation* 2009, **16**(2):121-137.

23. Investigators B: **Influence of Diabetes on 5-Year Mortality and Morbidity in a Randomized Trial Comparing CABG and PTCA in Patients With Multivessel Disease The Bypass Angioplasty Revascularization Investigation (BARI).** *Circulation* 1997, **96**(6):1761-1769.

24. Féart C, Samieri C, Alles B, Barberger-Gateau P: **Potential benefits of adherence to the Mediterranean diet on cognitive health.** *Proceedings of the Nutrition Society* 2013, **72**(01):140-152.

25. Cook NR, Cutler JA, Obarzanek E, Buring JE, Rexrode KM, Kumanyika SK, Appel LJ, Whelton PK: **Long term effects of dietary sodium reduction on cardiovascular disease outcomes: observational follow-up of the trials of hypertension prevention (TOHP).** *Bmj* 2007, **334**(7599):885.

26. Cecchini M, Sassi F, Lauer JA, Lee YY, Guajardo-Barron V, Chisholm D: **Tackling of unhealthy diets, physical inactivity, and obesity: health effects and cost-effectiveness.** *The Lancet* 2010, **376**(9754):1775-1784.

27. Hagströmer M, Troiano RP, Sjöström M, Berrigan D: **Levels and patterns of objectively assessed physical activity—a comparison between Sweden and the United States.** *American journal of epidemiology* 2010:kwq069.

28. Chaloupka FJ, Straif K, Leon ME: **Effectiveness of tax and price policies in tobacco control.** *Tobacco Control* 2010:tc. 2010.039982.

29. Schaap MM, Kunst AE, Leinsalu M, Regidor E, Ekholm O, Dzurova D, Helmert U, Klumbiene J, Santana P, Mackenbach JP: **Effect of nationwide tobacco control policies on smoking cessation in high and low educated groups in 18 European countries.** *Tobacco Control* 2008, **17**(4):248-255.

30. Wolf-Maier K, Cooper RS, Kramer H, Banegas JR, Giampaoli S, Joffres MR, Poulter N, Primatesta P, Stegmayr B, Thamm M: **Hypertension treatment and control in five European countries, Canada, and the United States.** *Hypertension* 2004, **43**(1):10-17.

31. Heuschmann PU, Kircher J, Nowe T, Dittrich R, Reiner Z, Cifkova R, Malojcic B, Mayer O, Bruthans J, Wloch-Kopec D: **Control of main risk factors after ischaemic stroke across Europe: data from the stroke-specific module of the EUROASPIRE III survey.** *European journal of preventive cardiology* 2015, **22**(10):1354-1362.

32.   Krishnamurthi RV, Moran AE, Feigin VL, Barker-Collo S, Norrving B, Mensah GA, Taylor S, Naghavi M, Forouzanfar MH, Nguyen G: **Stroke prevalence, mortality and disability-adjusted life years in adults aged 20-64 years in 1990-2013: data from the global burden of disease 2013 study**. *Neuroepidemiology* 2015, **45**(3):190-202.

33.   Pomerleau J, Lock K, McKee M: **The burden of cardiovascular disease and cancer attributable to low fruit and vegetable intake in the European Union: differences between old and new Member States**. *Public health nutrition* 2006, **9**(05):575-583.

34.   Kelly BB, Fuster V: **Promoting Cardiovascular Health in the Developing World:: A Critical Challenge to Achieve Global Health**: National Academies Press; 2010.

35.   Leal J, Luengo-Fernández R, Gray A, Petersen S, Rayner M: **Economic burden of cardiovascular diseases in the enlarged European Union**. *European heart journal* 2006, **27**(13):1610-1619.

36.   Ploug UJ: **The cost of diabetes-related complications: registry-based analysis of days absent from work**. *Economics Research International* 2013, **2013**.

37.   Løgstrup S, O'Kelly S: **European cardiovascular disease statistics: 2012 edition**. *Brussels, Belgium: European Heart Network* 2012.

38.   Diez Roux AV: **Investigating neighborhood and area effects on health**. *American journal of public health* 2001, **91**(11):1783-1789.

39.   Phelan JC, Link BG, Diez-Roux A, Kawachi I, Levin B: **"Fundamental causes" of social inequalities in mortality: a test of the theory**. *Journal of health and social behavior* 2004, **45**(3):265-285.

40.   Phelan JC, Link BG, Tehranifar P: **Social conditions as fundamental causes of health inequalities theory, evidence, and policy implications**. *Journal of health and social behavior* 2010, **51**(1 suppl):S28-S40.

41.   Diez Roux AV, Mair C: **Neighborhoods and health**. *Annals of the New York Academy of Sciences* 2010, **1186**(1):125-145.

42.   Link BG, Phelan J: **Social conditions as fundamental causes of disease**. *Journal of health and social behavior* 1995:80-94.

43.   Roux AVD: **Residential environments and cardiovascular risk**. *Journal of Urban Health* 2003, **80**(4):569-589.

44.   Roux AVD: **Estimating neighborhood health effects: the challenges of causal inference in a complex world**. *Social science & medicine* 2004, **58**(10):1953-1960.

45.   Roux AVD, Kershaw K, Lisabeth L: **Neighborhoods and cardiovascular risk: beyond individual-level risk factors**. *Current Cardiovascular Risk Reports* 2008, **2**(3):175-180.

46.   Roux AVD, Merkin SS, Arnett D, Chambless L, Massing M, Nieto FJ, Sorlie P, Szklo M, Tyroler HA, Watson RL: **Neighborhood of residence and incidence of coronary heart disease**. *New England Journal of Medicine* 2001, **345**(2):99-106.

47.   Lisabeth L: **Neighborhoods and Cardiovascular Risk: Beyond Individual-Level Risk Factors**. 2008.

48.   Association AD: **Diagnosis and classification of diabetes mellitus**. *Diabetes care* 2010, **33**(Supplement 1):S62-S69.

49.   de Ferranti SD, de Boer IH, Fonseca V, Fox CS, Golden SH, Lavie CJ, Magge SN, Marx N, McGuire DK, Orchard TJ: **Type 1 Diabetes Mellitus and Cardiovascular Disease A Scientific Statement From the American Heart Association and American Diabetes Association**. *Circulation* 2014, **130**(13):1110-1130.

50.   Vos T, Flaxman AD, Naghavi M, Lozano R, Michaud C, Ezzati M, Shibuya K, Salomon JA, Abdalla S, Aboyans V: **Years lived with disability (YLDs) for 1160 sequelae of 289 diseases and injuries 1990–2010: a systematic analysis for the Global Burden of Disease Study 2010**. *The Lancet* 2013, **380**(9859):2163-2196.

51. Maahs DM, West NA, Lawrence JM, Mayer-Davis EJ: **Epidemiology of type 1 diabetes**. *Endocrinology and metabolism clinics of North America* 2010, **39**(3):481-497.

52. Jonasson JM, Ye W, Sparén P, Apelqvist J, Nyrén O, Brismar K: **Risks of Nontraumatic Lower-Extremity Amputations in Patients with Type 1 Diabetes A population-based cohort study in Sweden**. *Diabetes Care* 2008, **31**(8):1536-1540.

53. Nyström T, Holzmann MJ, Eliasson B, Kuhl J, Sartipy U: **Glycemic control in type 1 diabetes and long-term risk of cardiovascular events or death after coronary artery bypass grafting**. *Journal of the American College of Cardiology* 2015, **66**(5):535-543.

54. Lim SS, Vos T, Flaxman AD, Danaei G, Shibuya K, Adair-Rohani H, AlMazroa MA, Amann M, Anderson HR, Andrews KG: **A comparative risk assessment of burden of disease and injury attributable to 67 risk factors and risk factor clusters in 21 regions, 1990–2010: a systematic analysis for the Global Burden of Disease Study 2010**. *The lancet* 2013, **380**(9859):2224-2260.

55. Schnell O, Cappuccio F, Genovese S, Standl E, Valensi P, Ceriello A: **Type 1 diabetes and cardiovascular disease**. *Cardiovasc Diabetol* 2013, **12**(1):156.

56. Deshpande AD, Harris-Hayes M, Schootman M: **Epidemiology of diabetes and diabetes-related complications**. *Physical therapy* 2008, **88**(11):1254-1264.

57. Kawachi I, Kennedy BP: **The health of nations**. *Why inequality is harmful to your health* 2002.

58. Walker AC, Aspalter C: **Securing the future for old age in Europe**. *Securing the Future for Old Age in Europe (Alan C Walker and Christian Aspalter, Casa Verde, Tapei, 2008)* 2008.

59. Ahgren B: **Health Care Delivery System: Sweden**. *The Wiley Blackwell Encyclopedia of Health, Illness, Behavior, and Society* 2014.

60. Burström B: **Increasing inequalities in health care utilisation across income groups in Sweden during the 1990s?** *Health policy* 2002, **62**(2):117-129.

61. Burstrom B: **Will Swedish healthcare reforms affect equity?** *BMJ British medical journal* 2010, **340**(7737):79-80.

62. Burström B: **Market-oriented, demand-driven health care reforms and equity in health and health care utilization in Sweden**. *International Journal of Health Services* 2009, **39**(2):271-285.

63. Dahlgren G: **Neoliberal Reforms in Swedish primary health care: for whom and for what purpose?** *International Journal of Health Services* 2008, **38**(4):697-715.

64. Barr D, Fenton L, Blane D: **The claim for patient choice and equity**. *Journal of medical ethics* 2008, **34**(4):271-274.

65. Fotaki M, Roland M, Boyd A, McDonald R, Scheaff R, Smith L: **What benefits will choice bring to patients? Literature review and assessment of implications**. *Journal of Health Services Research & Policy* 2008, **13**(3):178-184.

66. Danielsson M, Talbäck M: **Public health: An overview Health in Sweden: The National Public Health Report 2012. Chapter 1**. *Scandinavian journal of public health* 2012, **40**(9 suppl):6-22.

67. Organization WH: **Global action plan for the prevention and control of noncommunicable diseases 2013-2020**. 2013.

68. Pickett KE, Pearl M: **Multilevel analyses of neighbourhood socioeconomic context and health outcomes: a critical review**. *Journal of epidemiology and community health* 2001, **55**(2):111-122.

69. Anderson RT, Sorlie P, Backlund E, Johnson N, Kaplan GA: **Mortality effects of community socioeconomic status**. *Epidemiology* 1997, **8**(1):42-47.

70. Marmot M: **Social determinants of health inequalities**. *The Lancet* 2005, **365**(9464):1099-1104.

71.   Sampson RJ, Morenoff JD, Gannon-Rowley T: **Assessing" neighborhood effects": Social processes and new directions in research.** *Annual review of sociology* 2002:443-478.

72.   Messer LC, Laraia BA, Kaufman JS, Eyster J, Holzman C, Culhane J, Elo I, Burke JG, O'campo P: **The development of a standardized neighborhood deprivation index.** *Journal of Urban Health* 2006, **83**(6):1041-1062.

73.   Sundquist K, Malmström M, Johansson S, Sundquist J: **Care need index, a useful tool for the distribution of primary health care resources.** *Journal of epidemiology and community health* 2003, **57**(5):347-352.

74.   Payne RA: **UK indices of multiple deprivation-a way to make comparisons across constituent countries easier.** *Health* 2012, 4(13.5):13.15.

75.   Lahti Edmark H: **Storstad i rörelse: kunskapsöversikt över utvärderingar av storstadspolitikens lokala utvecklingsavtal: slutbetänkande.** *Statens offentliga utredningar* 2005.

76.   Kim ES, Hawes AM, Smith J: **Perceived neighbourhood social cohesion and myocardial infarction.** *Journal of epidemiology and community health* 2014:jech-2014-204009.

77.   Stjärne MK, Fritzell J, De Leon AP, Hallqvist J, Group SS: **Neighborhood socioeconomic context, individual income and myocardial infarction.** *Epidemiology* 2006, **17**(1):14-23.

78.   Kjærulff T, Schipperijn J, Gislason G, Ersbøll A: **Association between Neighborhood Socioeconomic Position and Risk of Incident Acute Myocardial Infarction in Denmark: A Spatial Analysis Approach.** *International Journal of Epidemiology* 2015, **44**(suppl 1):i278-i279.

79.   Sundquist K, Theobald H, Yang M, Li X, Johansson S-E, Sundquist J: **Neighborhood violent crime and unemployment increase the risk of coronary heart disease: a multilevel study in an urban setting.** *Social science & medicine* 2006, **62**(8):2061-2071.

80.   Lawlor DA, Davey Smith G, Patel R, Ebrahim S: **Life-course socioeconomic position, area deprivation, and coronary heart disease: findings from the British Women's Heart and Health Study.** *American journal of public health* 2005, **95**(1):91-97.

81.   Aslanyan S, Weir CJ, Lees KR, Reid JL, McInnes GT: **Effect of area-based deprivation on the severity, subtype, and outcome of ischemic stroke.** *Stroke* 2003, **34**(11):2623-2628.

82.   Pujades-Rodriguez M, Timmis A, Stogiannis D, Rapsomaniki E, Denaxas S, Shah A, Feder G, Kivimaki M, Hemingway H: **Socioeconomic deprivation and the incidence of 12 cardiovascular diseases in 1.9 million women and men: implications for risk prediction and prevention.** *PloS one* 2014, **9**(8):e104671.

83.   Ferguson HJM, Nightingale P, Pathak R, Jayatunga AP: **The influence of socio-economic deprivation on rates of major lower limb amputation secondary to peripheral arterial disease.** *European Journal of Vascular and Endovascular Surgery* 2010, **40**(1):76-80.

84.   Bihan H, Laurent S, Sass C, Nguyen G, Huot C, Moulin JJ, Guegen R, Le Toumelin P, Le Clésiau H, La Rosa E: **Association Among Individual Deprivation, Glycemic Control, and Diabetes Complications The EPICES score.** *Diabetes care* 2005, **28**(11):2680-2685.

85.   Matteucci E, Giampietro O: **Epidemiology of cardiovascular disease in patients with type 1 diabetes: European perspective.** *Experimental and clinical endocrinology & diabetes: official journal, German Society of Endocrinology [and] German Diabetes Association* 2014, **122**(4):208-214.

86.   Roper NA, Bilous RW, Kelly WF, Unwin NC, Connolly VM: **Excess mortality in a population with diabetes and the impact of material deprivation: longitudinal, population based study.** *Bmj* 2001, **322**(7299):1389-1393.

87.   Robinson N, Lloyd C, Stevens L: **Social deprivation and mortality in adults with diabetes mellitus.** *Diabetic medicine* 1998, **15**(3):205-212.
88.   Rawshani A, Svensson A-M, Rosengren A, Eliasson B, Gudbjörnsdottir S: **Impact of Socioeconomic Status on Cardiovascular Disease and Mortality in 24,947 Individuals With Type 1 Diabetes.** *Diabetes care* 2015, **38**(8):1518-1527.
89.   Sweden S: **Official statistics of Sweden.** *Upp till* 2015, **18**.
90.   Wettermark B, Hammar N, MichaelFored C, Leimanis A, Otterblad Olausson P, Bergman U, Persson I, Sundström A, Westerholm B, Rosén M: **The new Swedish Prescribed Drug Register—opportunities for pharmacoepidemiological research and experience from the first six months.** *Pharmacoepidemiology and drug safety* 2007, **16**(7):726-735.
91.   Ludvigsson JF, Otterblad-Olausson P, Pettersson BU, Ekbom A: **The Swedish personal identity number: possibilities and pitfalls in healthcare and medical research.** *European journal of epidemiology* 2009, **24**(11):659-667.
92.   Ludvigsson JF, Andersson E, Ekbom A, Feychting M, Kim J-L, Reuterwall C, Heurgren M, Olausson PO: **External review and validation of the Swedish national inpatient register.** *BMC public health* 2011, **11**(1):1.
93.   Johansson LA, Westerling R: **Comparing Swedish hospital discharge records with death certificates: implications for mortality statistics.** *International journal of epidemiology* 2000, **29**(3):495-502.
94.   Andersson R: **'Divided cities' as a policy-based notion in Sweden.** *Housing studies* 1999, **14**(5):601-624.
95.   Andersson R, Bråmå Å, Holmqvist E: **Counteracting segregation: Swedish policies and experiences.** *Housing studies* 2010, **25**(2):237-256.
96.   Nathan DM, Bebu I, Braffett BH, Orchard TJ, Cowie CC, Lopes-Virella M, Schutta M, Lachin JM, Control D, Trial C *et al*: **Risk Factors for Cardiovascular Disease in Type 1 Diabetes.** *Diabetes* 2016:db151517.
97.   Mozaffarian D, Benjamin EJ, Go AS, Arnett DK, Blaha MJ, Cushman M, Das SR, de Ferranti S, Després J-P, Fullerton HJ: **Executive Summary: Heart Disease and Stroke Statistics—2016 Update A Report From the American Heart Association.** *Circulation* 2016, **133**(4):447-454.
98.   Board SDI: **Personal Data Act (1998: 204).** In.; 2012.
99.   Hanson MA, Gluckman PD: **Developmental processes and the induction of cardiovascular function: conceptual aspects.** *The Journal of physiology* 2005, **565**(1):27-34.
100.   Bo Burström KB DC: **Livsvillkor, levnadsvanor och hälsa i Stockholms län. 2014.** In.: Karolinska Institutet; 2014.
101.   Akhavan S, Tillgren P, Aytar O, Bogg L, Söderlund A: **Practice and Policy in Promoting Health and Equity–experiences from a national project in primary health care in Sweden.** In: *22nd IUHPE World Conference on Health Promotion, CURITIBA, BRAZIL: 2016*; 2016.
102.   Andersson R: **'Breaking Segregation'—Rhetorical Construct or Effective Policy? The Case of the Metropolitan Development Initiative in Sweden.** *Urban Studies* 2006, **43**(4):787-799.
103.   Near AM, Blackman K, Currie LM, Levy DT: **Sweden SimSmoke: the effect of tobacco control policies on smoking and snus prevalence and attributable deaths.** *The European Journal of Public Health* 2014, **24**(3):451-458.
104.   Rosén M: **Price and health policy in Sweden—A critical review.** *Health Policy* 1989, **12**(3):263-274.
105.   Cisneros Örnberg J: **The Europeanization of Swedish alcohol policy.** 2009.
106.   Konbérg B: **Tobacco control in Sweden.** *Tobacco and health* 1995:107.
107.   Saffer H, Chaloupka F: **The effect of tobacco advertising bans on tobacco consumption.** *Journal of health economics* 2000, **19**(6):1117-1137.

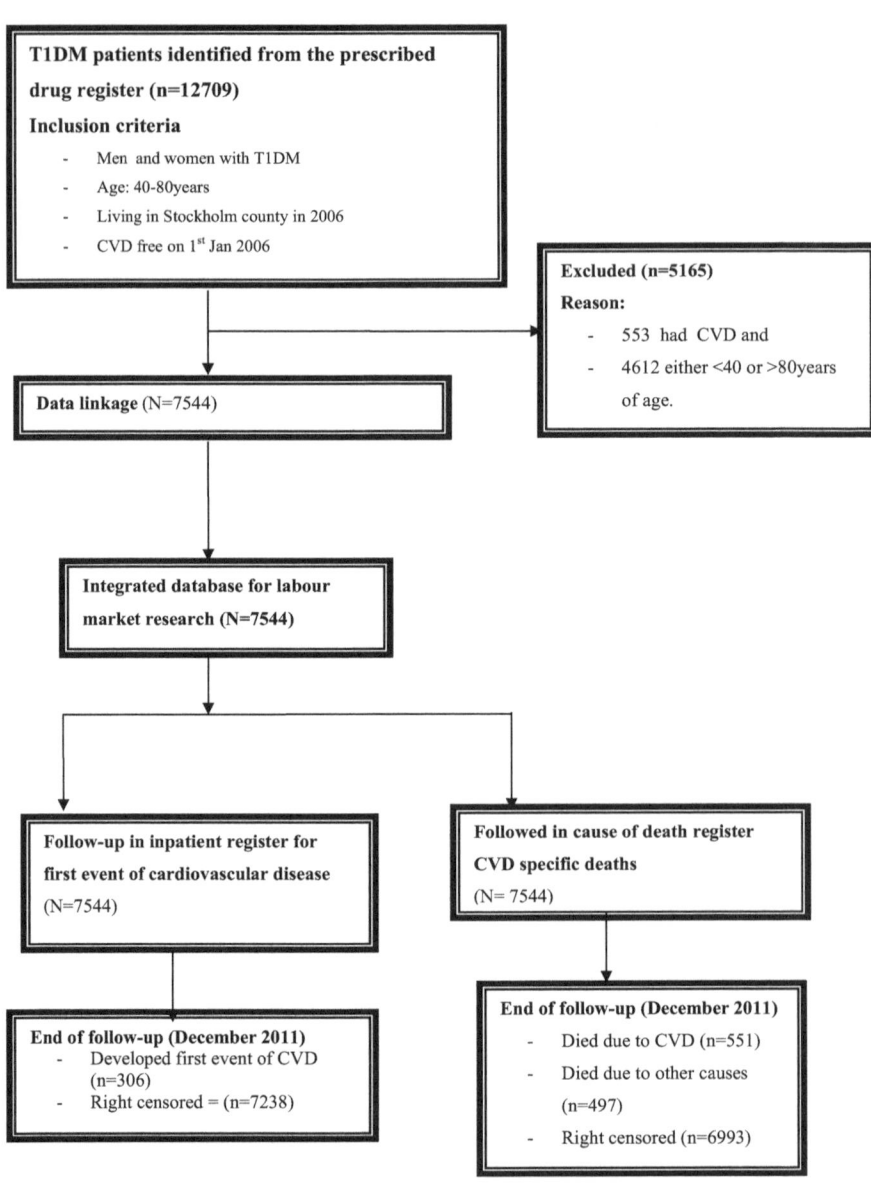

Appendix 1: Flow Diagram of data linkage and follow-up

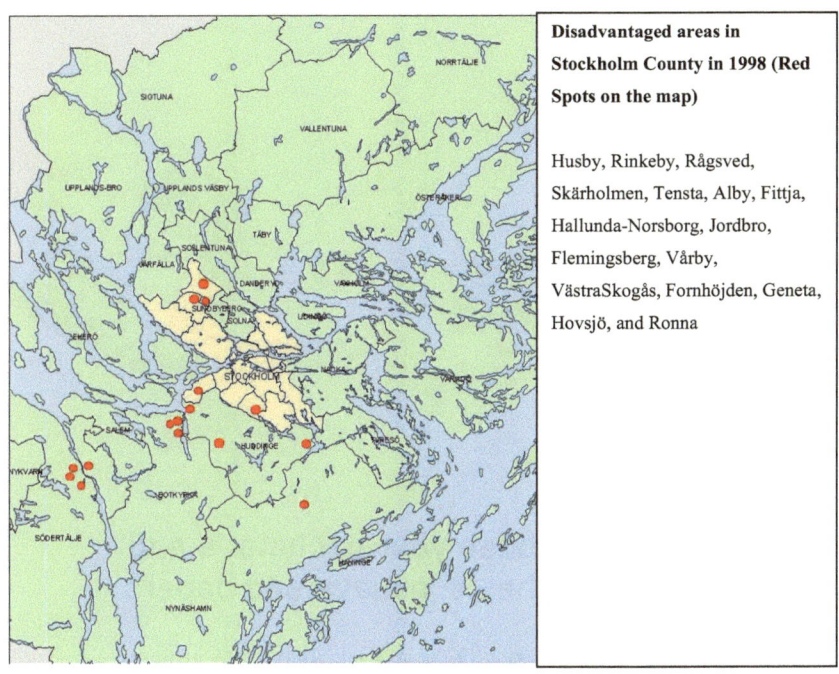

	Disadvantaged areas in Stockholm County in 1998 (Red Spots on the map)
	Husby, Rinkeby, Rågsved, Skärholmen, Tensta, Alby, Fittja, Hallunda-Norsborg, Jordbro, Flemingsberg, Vårby, VästraSkogås, Fornhöjden, Geneta, Hovsjö, and Ronna

Appendix 2: Map of Stockholm County showing disadvantaged areas

Source: Bo Burström KB DC: Livsvillkor, levnadsvanor och hälsa i Stockholms län. 2014. **In.: Karolinska Institutet; 2014.**

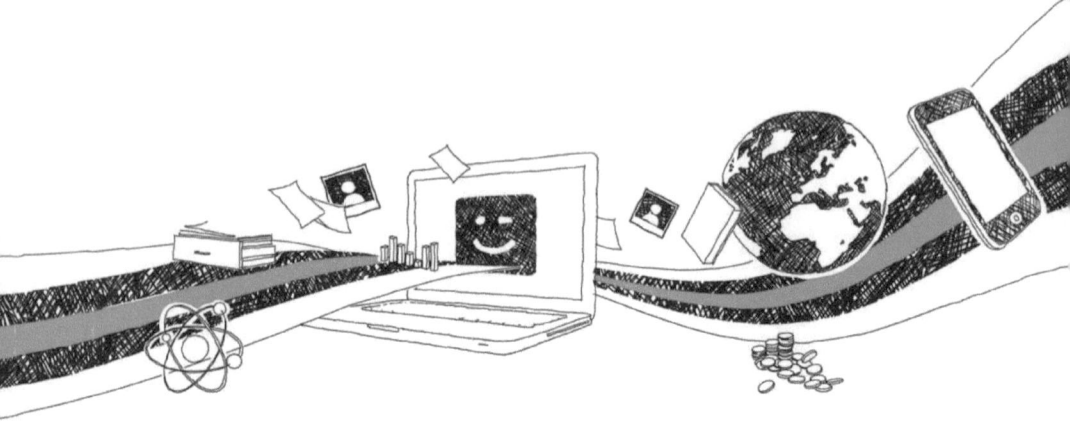
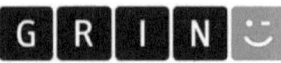